Health Benefits

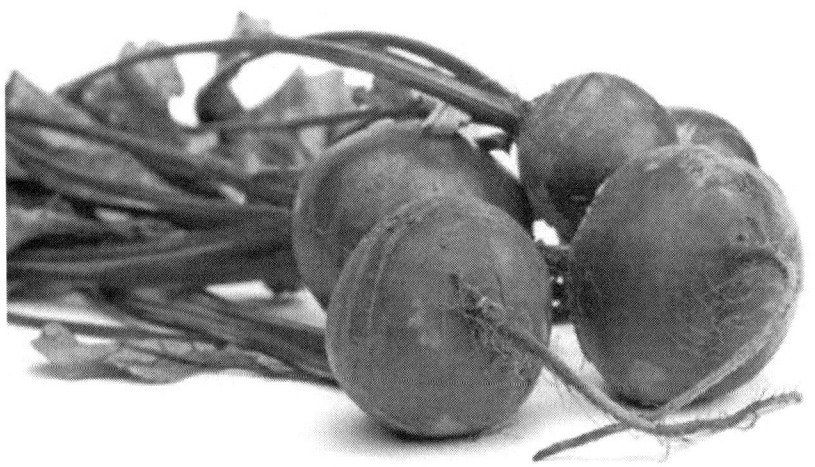

Health Learning Series
M. Usman
Mendon Cottage Books
JD-Biz Publishing

All Rights Reserved.

No part of this publication may be reproduced in any form or by any means, including scanning, photocopying, or otherwise without prior written permission from JD-Biz Corp Copyright © 2014

All Images Licensed by Fotolia and 123RF.

Disclaimer

The information is this book is provided for informational purposes only. It is not intended to be used and medical advice or a substitute for proper medical treatment by a qualified health care provider. The information is believed to be accurate as presented based on research by the author.

The contents have not been evaluated by the U.S. Food and Drug Administration or any other Government or Health Organization and the contents in this book are not to be used to treat cure or prevent disease.

The author or publisher is not responsible for the use or safety of any diet, procedure or treatment mentioned in this book. The author or publisher is not responsible for errors or omissions that may exist.

Warning

The Book is for informational purposes only and before taking on any diet, treatment or medical procedure, it is recommended to consult with your primary health care provider.

Check out some of the other Healthy Gardening Series books at Amazon.com

Gardening Series on Amazon

Check out some of the other Health Learning Series books at Amazon.com

Health Learning Series on Amazon

Table of Contents

Preface 4
Getting Started 5
Chapter # 1: Intro 5
Chapter # 2: Nutritional Worth 9
Chapter # 3: Selection & Storage 14
Health Benefits 16
Chapter # 1: Cardiovascular Health 16
Chapter # 2: Lowers Risk of Dementia 18
Chapter # 3: Improves Athletic Performance 20
Chapter # 4: Good for the Skin & Hair 22
Recipes 24
Chapter # 1: Beetroot and Walnut Salad 24
Chapter # 2: Tandoori Cutlets with Beetroot Raita 26
Chapter # 3: Beetroot Hummus 28
Conclusion 29
References 30
Author Bio 31

Preface

Beetroot, sometimes also referred to as the beet, is a part of a vegetable that is gaining immense fame in health-aware populations due to its lengthy list of nutritious benefits. Beetroots and their products like juices & concentrates have countless benefits, some of which include the restoration of body's normal functions like blood pressure, blood flow, and athletic performance. More and more pharmaceutical companies are now using compounds extracted from beetroot in their products due to their superior antioxidant, refreshing and cardiovascular benefit inducing properties.

Beetroots have, for long, been in use by ancient civilizations due to their refreshing and detoxification qualities. The rich purple pigment in beetroots is one of the most nutritious components of the vegetable and is known to suppress the development of deadly diseases like Alzheimer's and cancer.

Read on, and find out more.

Getting Started

Chapter # 1: Intro

To understand beetroot, one must first grasp the concept of a taproot. Taproot is the largest and most dominant root in plants; it is straight and very thick in appearance and grows directly into the ground. For example, the orange part of a carrot that is mostly eaten is its taproot; similarly, the beetroot is the taproot portion of the beet plant attached to the green leaves of the vegetable.

Beetroot, botanically called Beta Vulgaris, is also known by names like table beet, red beet, golden beet and garden beet, but most people almost always remove the "root" plant of the word and call it by the name beet. The most common type of beet is of a deep purple color but nonetheless, white, yellow and rainbow colored varieties are also available in vegetable markets. Beetroots might look tough in texture, but they are not that hard and the smallest puncture can cause the red-purple pigments (known to be the epicenter of beet's health-promoting properties) to bleed. Beets' sweet taste is related to its high sugar content which is one of the main reasons for its high popularity. The pigments in beet are not only highly water soluble but are also temperature sensitive, therefore, it is necessary that beets are treated with care; this has been explained in the coming chapters.

Raw beetroots are crunchy in texture and turn soft and buttery when they are cooked. Apart from being boiled and baked, the roots are also a primary component in many salads. Another very common form of the vegetable is its juice, which is naturally sweet in taste and packs a plethora of benefits for the body. Soups made from beets, like cold borsch, are extremely popular in Europe. Pickled beets are also becoming very common in Australia and New Zealand as more and more people like to have them with hamburgers.

The origin of beets can be traced as far back as 4000 years ago when the ancient Babylonians started to use it for their health benefits. But, beets weren't truly commercialized until the Romans, like many other vegetables, started to cultivate it. The tribes that invaded Rome were responsible for further spreading of the vegetable throughout Northern Europe where they first found their use as animal fodder and then finally human consumption. By the 19th Century, beets held great commercial value as it had been discovered that sugar can be extracted from them. The first sugar factory for this particular extraction was established in Poland. This particular quality was extremely beneficial for Napoleonic France when the British blockaded the country's sugar supply. During the same time period, beets made their way into the United States where they now flourish. The leading commercial producers of beets in the modern world include Russia, USA, Poland, France and Germany.

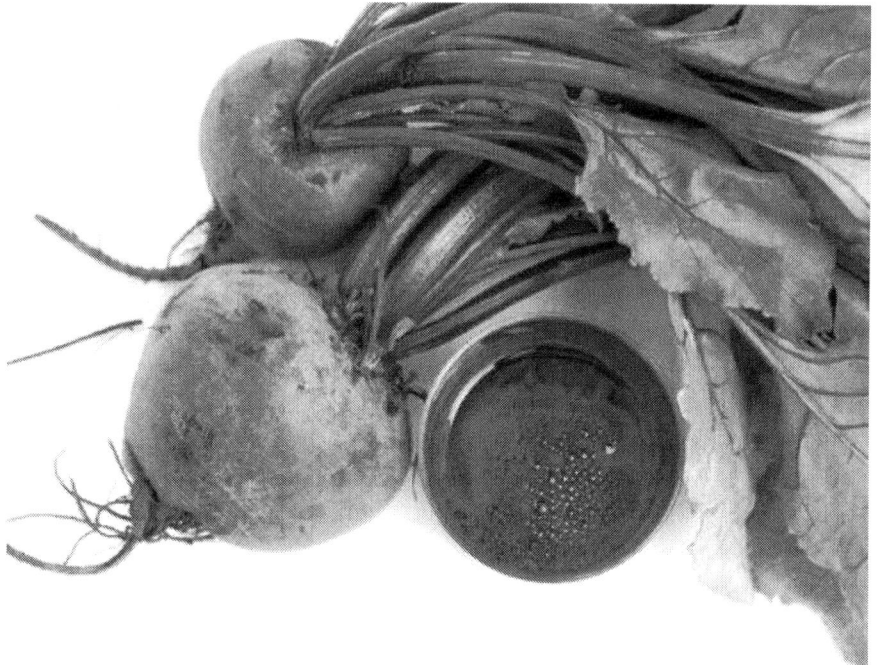

The health benefits of beetroot are:

- Exhibiting anti-cancer activity - beetroot contains a compound betacyanin that can detoxify the body of hazardous chemicals and prevent the formation of tumors in the body. This particular compound is known to have a marked effect on cancers including, lung, skin, leukemia, breast, testicular, and especially stomach cancer.

- Preventing cell damage – beetroot contains a pigment that is a known anti-inflammatory, fungicidal and antioxidant. This prevents the cells from DNA damage and scavenging from free radicals; it also reduces oxidative stress which is becoming increasingly common in the new generation.

- Solvent of inorganic calcium in the body – inorganic calcium deposits are one of the major reasons for chronic diseases that include, kidney stones, arthritis and varicose veins.

- Improving digestive health – beetroot has the ability to deal with digestive problems like fat digestion and alterations in the body's metabolism.

- Aiding pregnant women – beetroot is very beneficial for pregnant women as it eliminates various birth defects due to its high folic acid content. It also aids in tissue growth and improved development of the baby's spinal cord.

- Beneficial for the eyes – beetroot packs a class of health-promoting compounds including carotenoids that are good for the retinal part of the eye. Raw beetroot is the best way to add these compounds to the system.

- Improves physical activity- beetroot aids in reducing negative effects of exercise, both during and after. It enhances the body's stamina and persistence which is a good source of motivation for many.

- Better blood flow – drinking a single glass of beetroot aids in blood flow to parts of the body that helps prevent ailments like dementia. Beetroot performs this task by widening the blood vessels and reducing the extra use of oxygen by muscles during physical activity.

- Improved blood supply – beetroot is rich in both iron and antioxidants that makes the perfect recipe for proper blood supply.

The iron content is useful for people with anemia or low hemoglobin; it facilitates the absorption of iron into the bloodstream, as a result of which there is an increase in the blood count and oxygen carrying capacity of the red blood cells. Nitrates are another class of compounds in beetroot that improve the blood flow in the heart and muscles; they achieve this by opening up blood vessels throughout the body.

This is the just the beginning, as there are many other benefits of beetroots that will be tracked and tackled throughout every chapter of this book. For now, you will be taken through the nutritional details of the very heartwarming vegetable that is beetroot.

Chapter # 2: Nutritional Worth

Beetroots are of exceptional nutritional worth. Did you know that garden beets (one's that are consumed most often) are very low in calories? There are only 45 kcal in a 100 g serving of beets and that too, with no cholesterol. The benefits of beetroots are mainly owed to its unique vitamin, mineral and fiber content. One phytochemical compound in beetroot that is worth mentioning is *glycine betaine;* this particular phytochemical controls the levels of a highly toxic compound that causes plaque formation in blood vessels, and you know what plaque leads to: cardiovascular diseases including coronary heart disease, vascular diseases and the infamous stroke.

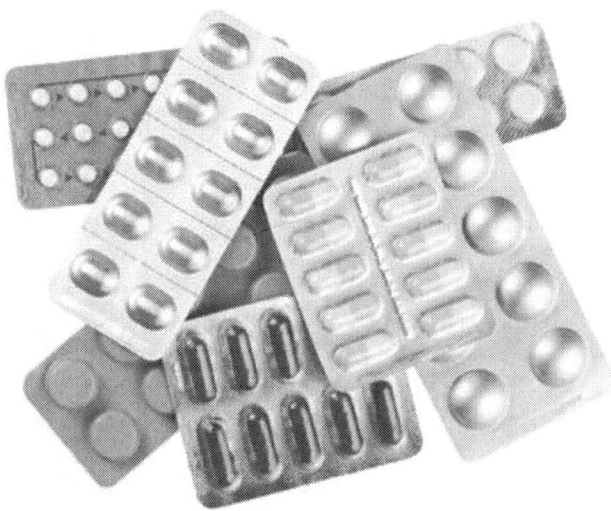

Raw beets can also fulfill 27% of the body's daily requirement of Folate. Folate are vital for correct DNA synthesis in the body as well as for neural tubes of a baby, but extensive cooking can significantly deplete the level of folate in beets, so emphasis must be laid on the "raw" part of the beets. Beets are also a great source of vitamin C especially the top part. A 100 g of beet greens can provide 50% of the daily amount of RDA. Vitamin C, as most people know it, is a strong antioxidant that prevents the body from scavengers, like oxidants, that ultimately play a hand in cancer development.

Additionally, beetroots can also provide the body with vitamin A and other antioxidants that are essential for skin and oral health. The roots are a rich source of B-vitamins and minerals like iron, manganese, magnesium, copper and potassium which all play due roles in the maintenance of the human body.

A detailed account of the nutritional wellness of **raw beets** is given in the following table. The amount taken is that of a single beet that weighs 82 grams and has a 2 inch diameter.

Calorie Information		
Nutrient	**Amount**	**% DV**
Total Calories	35.3 (148 kJ)	2%
From Carbohydrates	30.4 (127 kJ)	
From Fat	1.2 (5.0 kJ)	
From Proteins	3.6 (15.5 kJ)	
Carbohydrates		
Nutrient	**Amount**	**% DV**
Total Carbohydrates	7.8 g	9%
Dietary Fiber	2.3 g	9%
Starch	0.0 g	
Sugar	5.5 g	
Fats & Fatty Acids		
Nutrient	**Amount**	**% DV**
Total Fat	0.1 g	0%
Saturated Fat	0.0 g	0%
Mono-saturated Fat	0.0 g	
Polyunsaturated Fat	0.0 g	
Total Omega-3 Fatty acids	4.1 mg	
Total Omega-6 Fatty acids	45.1 mg	
Proteins		
Nutrient	**Amount**	**% DV**
Protein	1.3 g	3%
Vitamins		

Nutrient	Amount	% DV
Vitamin A	27.1 IU	1%
Vitamin C	4.0 mg	7%
Vitamin E	0.0 mg	0%
Vitamin K	0.2 mcg	0%
Thiamin	0.0 mg	2%
Riboflavin	0.0 mg	2%
Niacin	0.3 mg	1%
Vitamin B6	0.1 mg	3%
Folate	89.4 mcg	22%
Vitamin B12	0.0 mg	0%
Pantothenic Acid	0.1 mg	1%
Choline	4.9 mg	
Betaine	106 mg	
Minerals		
Nutrient	Amount	% DV
Calcium	13.1 mg	1%
Iron	0.7 mg	4%
Magnesium	18.9 mg	5%
Phosphorus	32.8 mg	3%
Potassium	267 mg	8%
Sodium	64.0 mg	3%
Zinc	0.3 mg	2%
Copper	0.1 mg	3%
Manganese	0.3 mg	13%
Selenium	0.6 mcg	1%

The following is a table stating the nutritional worth of **2 beets** that have been **cooked, boiled** and then finally **drained**. The diameter of each beet is 2 inches while the weight is 100 grams.

Calorie Information		
Nutrient	**Amount**	**% DV**
Total Calories	44.0 (184 kJ)	2%
From Carbohydrates	37.8 (158 kJ)	
From Fat	1.5 (6.3 kJ)	
From Proteins	4.7 (19.7 kJ)	
Carbohydrates		
Nutrient	**Amount**	**% DV**
Total Carbohydrates	10.0 g	3%
Dietary Fiber	2.0 g	8%
Starch	0.0 g	
Sugar	8.0 g	
Fats & Fatty Acids		
Nutrient	**Amount**	**% DV**
Total Fat	0.2 g	0%
Saturated Fat	0.0 g	0%
Mono-saturated Fat	0.0 g	
Polyunsaturated Fat	0.1 g	
Total Omega-3 Fatty acids	5.0 mg	
Total Omega-6 Fatty acids	58.0 mg	
Proteins		
Nutrient	**Amount**	**% DV**
Protein	1.7 g	3%
Vitamins		
Nutrient	**Amount**	**% DV**
Vitamin A	35.0 IU	1%
Vitamin C	3.6 mg	6%
Vitamin E	0.0 mg	0%
Vitamin K	0.2 mcg	0%
Thiamin	0.0 mg	2%
Riboflavin	0.0 mg	2%
Niacin	0.3 mg	2%

Vitamin B6	0.1 mg	3%
Folate	80.0 mcg	20%
Vitamin B12	0.0 mg	0%
Pantothenic Acid	0.1 mg	1%
Choline	6.3 mg	
Betaine	~	

Minerals		
Nutrient	**Amount**	**% DV**
Calcium	16.0 mg	2%
Iron	0.8 mg	4%
Magnesium	23.0 mg	6%
Phosphorus	38.0 mg	4%
Potassium	305 mg	9%
Sodium	77.0 mg	3%
Zinc	0.4 mg	2%
Copper	0.1 mg	4%
Manganese	0.3 mg	16%
Selenium	0.7 mcg	1%

You might have noticed that there are some differences between the two variants of beetroot; one that is most significant is the elimination of the phytochemical Betaine in the boiled version. Some other vitamins and minerals also are lost in the process but ultimately it depends on the benefits you want to reap. Boiling won't destroy the vegetable but if it is Betaine that you are looking for, then it is best to consume the vegetable raw.

Chapter # 3: Selection & Storage

Fresh beet season mostly runs through the months of June until October, but many markets import fresh beets from countries with opposite climate conditions to make it available year round. Moreover, beets are also available in canned form even though they are considered to be inferior.

When buying, choose beets that are small and firm when held and have a deep maroon coloring with unblemished skin & bright green leaves. Signs of wilting should be checked on the leaves as these indicate the freshness of the vegetable. Avoid beets that are large in size and have a hairy taproot, as all the roots that grow on the taproot are an indication of the ruggedness and agedness of the beet, which is not good. Most beets are 1-2 inches in diameter and any larger would have a tough, woody center. Also, smaller beets are more tender and sweeter in taste; exactly what you're looking for.

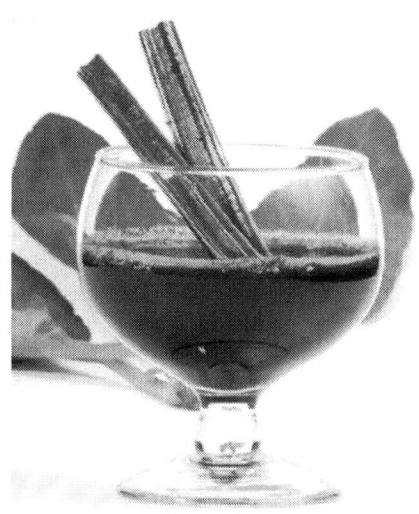

After purchasing, it's time to store them. To do so, trim the leaves of the beetroot, 2 inches from the taproot. The leaves will extract the moisture from the beetroot so trimming is absolutely necessary. Do not accidently or purposely trim the tail of the beetroot. Store the leaves in a separate bag if you wish to and if you do, use them within 2 days. The root bulbs should also be bagged and stored in a refrigerator's crisper drawer for 7 – 10 days. Cooked or canned beets can also be stored in a refrigerator and last for a week. Fresh cooked beets may be frozen for up to10 months. Remember to peel before freezing and use an airtight container, making sure that no air is left in the container.

Although beets are good to be eaten raw, they are generally boiled, steamed, baked, grilled, fried or cooked before consumption. Here are a few tricks that will come in handy when dealing with beetroots.

- Do not wash the beets roughly; you want the beet's skin to remain intact when cooking.
- To retain nutrients and color, boil, steam, or bake without peeling the beet. The skin will rub off easily under cold water after it has been cooked.
- When trimming, leave an inch of the leaf stems attached. The stem and root may be removed after cooking.
- If you must peel before cooking, use a swivel vegetable peeler rather than a paring knife.
- For best flavor, bake beets instead of steaming or boiling them. Wrap them in a foil so any staining can be avoided.

Health Benefits

Chapter # 1: Cardiovascular Health

The combination of organs in the body responsible for the efficient transportation of nutrients in and gaseous waste out of the body is known as the cardiovascular system. It is made up of mainly the heart, blood vessels and blood, but other lymphatic organs are also involved. The cardiovascular system is one of the foremost necessities for maintaining life and therefore should always be kept on a high note.

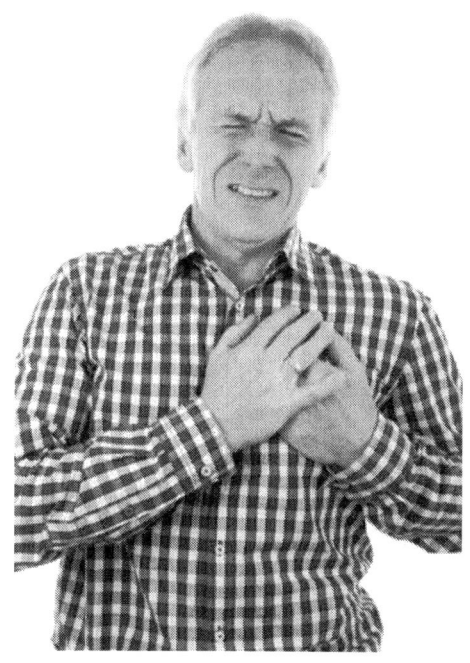

Beetroot and its products are a very good source of the chemical compound nitrate which can dramatically bring down high blood pressure. High blood pressure or hypertension is one of the main causes of diseases like strokes and heart attacks and researchers use it as a marker for more sophisticated cardiovascular diseases. Researchers from Queen Mary and University of London carried out a research showing that only a cup of beetroot juice was enough to lower blood pressure of patients suffering from hypertension, or more commonly, high blood pressure; the study was published in American Heart Association's Journal Hypertension. Just to be on the safe side, the scientists first carried out trials on rats and then confirmed their findings on 15 human subjects.

Where do nitrates come from? Just like every other mineral a plant acquires, nitrates also come from the soil and are sucked into the plant's system by their roots. Vegetables rich in nitrates include cabbage, lettuce, fennel and of course beetroot. It was believed by the researchers before carrying out the experiment that nitrates are converted into nitric oxide by the body, and it is this chemical that eases up the blood vessels. Eight females and seven males who had systolic blood pressure between 140 to 159 millimeters and no other medical problems were chosen for this study; they were not on any medication for their underlying disease. The participants were given a 250 ml drink of beetroot juice or water, which had a low amount of nitrate over a period of 24 hours and their blood pressure, was observed. Only 0.2 grams of nitrate (same as a large bowl of lettuce) was enough to make the participants feel a positive change in their bodies; this feeling was further reiterated by blood tests that showed a 10 point decrease in each participant's blood pressure levels (those who consumed beetroot juice and not water). The researchers were surprised by the large effect induced by such little amount of nitrates. The study showed that sufferers of hypertension can decrease their blood pressures simply by drinking beetroot juice.

About 16 million people in the UK alone suffer from hypertension. Many individuals aren't even aware of this fact and just keep on living their life, increasing their risk of experiencing a heart attack. All these people, and others, can make this little change to their lifestyle and be more protected from a cardiovascular nightmare.

Chapter # 2: Lowers Risk of Dementia

Dementia is a general term used to denote a combination of symptoms that all are related to cognitive decline such as memory loss, complexes, etc. It is not diagnosed clinically itself until a specific disease with same symptoms pop up. Under this umbrella, come problems related to memory, thinking and language. The most well-known disorder as a result of dementia is the Alzheimer's disease. The likelihood of a person developing dementia increases with one's age; light cognitive impairments soon become much more serious and lead to sophisticated diseases. There are many different categories of dementia but the symptoms are more or less the same:

- Difficulty in completing tasks,
- Recent memory loss,
- Difficulty in communicating,
- Disorientation,
- Mood swings,
- Personality changes and so on.

A study carried out by researchers from the Wake Forest University, USA has showed that beetroot juice had the ability to combat the onset of dementia. This was a small study targeting elders, 16 to be exact. The participants were each given a diet which was either high or low in nitrates for 4 days. It was previously known that nitrates widen up the blood vessels to bring down high blood pressure but researchers were trying to find out whether it affects the brain as well. The blood flow of each of the subjects was measured as means to study the effectiveness of the drink.

The research was divided into two phases. The first phase aimed at finding out the time period after ingestion at which the nitrates were most effective at widening the blood vessels. Five adults of age 70 were chosen for this task and their blood was drained out in 0.5, 1, 2 & 3 hour intervals. In the main phase of the research the 16 adults recruited for the study were put through a 10 hour overnight fast before being divided into two groups; one group received a low nitrate diet while the other received a high nitrate diet i.e. beetroot juice. In addition, both the groups were also given breakfast, lunch and dinner with their own specialized diet. The high nitrate diet consisted of beetroot juice for breakfast, bananas for snacks and leafy vegetables rich in nitrates as other meals.

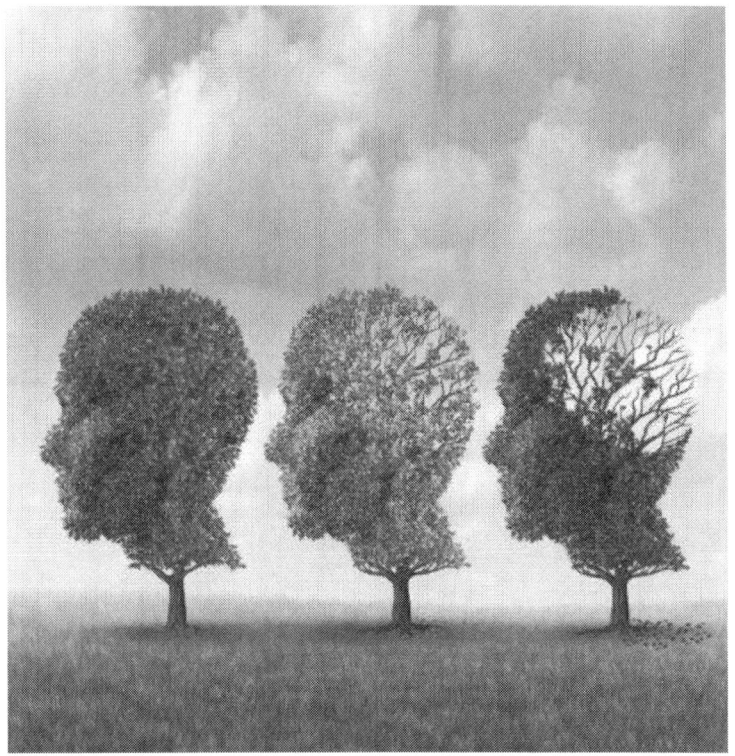

The researchers found out that the beetroot group had higher blood flow within the white matter of the lobes (frontal). This, in simple words, means adequate blood supply to parts of the brain that are infamous for running low on blood. The researchers were still left wondering how beetroot oxygenated the isolated parts of the brain but nonetheless it did work.

Chapter # 3: Improves Athletic Performance

Many athletes have started using beetroot supplements as means of improving their athletic performance. This approach seems to be a clear outcome of the fact that beetroot oxygenates the body therefore ensuring that enough oxygen is present in the muscles during a high intensity workout.

A US Study carried out by the St. Louis University in 2011 and presented to the American Dietetic Association, showed that when cooked beetroot were given to runners before a 5 km run, those who consumed beetroot had a 41 second advantage compared to those given a cranberry relish.

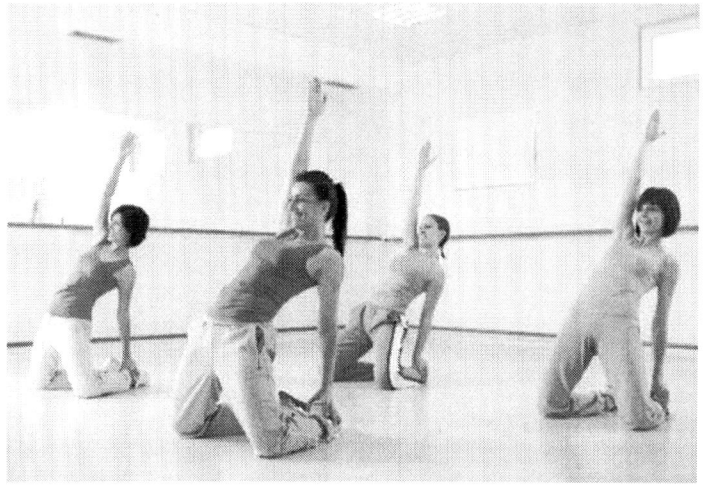

One study that aimed to find out beets' effectiveness for athletes showed that a 500 ml dose of beet juice each day increased the stamina by 15%. Since then, many medical researchers have been busy trying to find out more manageable methods to incorporate beetroots into the daily regimen. As juicing 3 to 5 beetroots every morning is a time consuming and sometimes messy task, alternatives such as powders and concentrated extracts are being introduced into the market. Researchers at the University of Exeter have already shown that concentrated beet juice is similar to fresh juice in increasing the time before an athlete reaches exhaustion. However, the same cannot be said about beet powder as results are still to come out for those tests.

Dosage - Researchers have showed that doses up to 600 ml had significant benefits for athletes but doubling the dose had no beneficial effect. Doses at 300 ml also showed improved performances so if you're starting out, 300 ml will be a good way to get the body adjusted for bigger doses.

Raw or cooked - Studies have already shown that cooking will drain out nitrates in vegetables like beets. This is why juicing or concentrating raw beet extracts are still the given preference when it comes to ingesting beets; one of the reason beets are included in salads. However, some people think that light steaming of the vegetable may actually make its vitamins easier to acquire.

Ingest it fast or slow – The nitrates in beets are first converted into nitrite by a process that goes on in our saliva. This is a vital step in the whole conversion and should be given due importance. This conversion takes time so therefore; use of toothpaste or other washing material soon after consuming beetroot juice may hinder the ability of the body to reap the full number of benefits. Thus, it follows that beetroot juice must be ingested slowly so the body could get more out of it.

Will it work – Just like all supplements; every person will have a unique response to the performance enhancing qualities of beets. The research at the University of Exeter stated that there were a number of "non-responders" in the study; these individuals weren't able to gain any benefit from the juice even at high doses. This behavior was explained by tight scrutiny in a scientific environment, which in the real world is not possible. Still, one should consider the possibility of beetroot not working and therefore should have an alternate as well.

One thing that should be kept in mind is moderation. Researchers have stressed out this point and have stated that consuming too much beetroot won't do well for the body; in-fact it would result in digestive distress which is no good for an athlete who has to run a mile in minutes.

Chapter # 4: Good for the Skin & Hair

Beetroot is beneficial for all parts of the body, including the skin. It was believed in Greek mythology that Aphrodite, the goddess of love, beauty & sexuality, drank beetroot juice to retain her beauty. Consumption of beetroot juice on a daily basis is very health-promoting for the body; it can cure & prevent from coming back, skin inflammations like boils and acne. Its anti-inflammatory content prevents any unnecessary outbursts like pimples. Beetroot juice achieves such effectiveness by purifying blood from within the body and cleansing it of excess toxins and water and as a result a healthy glow is imparted to a person's face. Furthermore, applying beet juice to the skin can keep it supple and hydrated. Regular consumption will give the face a glowing completion by removal of deal cells from the skin and replacing it with new ones. The powerful anti-oxidants also neutralize the effects of free-radicals that cause premature aging. Characteristics of premature ageing include wrinkles and lines on a person's face. A chemical lycopene also found in beetroots can maintain the elasticity of a person's skin and act as a natural sun-screen.

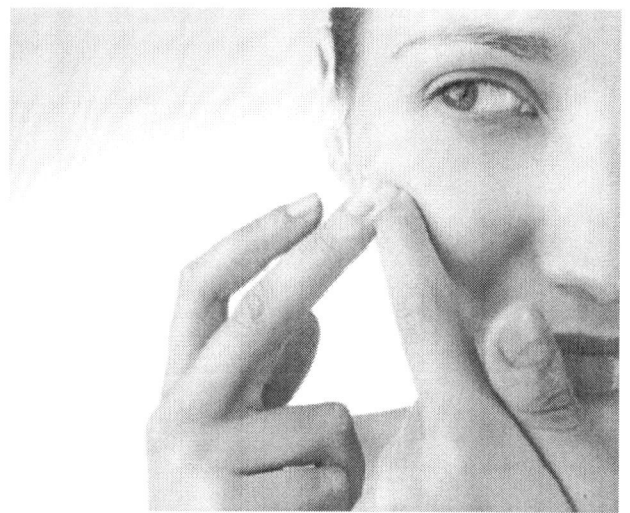

Beetroot can also be used as a natural beauty product; beetroot juice as mask can give the face a pinkish complexion. Just mix a tablespoon of beetroot juice with carrot juice; apply it all over your face with a cotton ball, leave it on for 10 minutes and wash off your face.

By now you must know that beetroot is excellent at opening up oxygen pathways in the body; one area whose health is directly related to blood circulation is the scalp. Beetroot juice not only increases blood flow in the scalp but also eliminates itchy scalps and dryness through its anti-pruritic properties. It destroys dead cells and moisturizes the scalp to alleviate dryness that is often accompanied with problems like dandruff. Beet juice can be mixed with vinegar to produce a solution that has the ability to cleanse the scalp of psoriasis. Furthermore, beetroot juice can be mixed with henna to create a natural dye. The dye would not only be chemical free, but would actually work and keep your hair healthy and beautiful. Also you can rinse your hair with diluted beetroot juice to get a reddish tint. Last but not the least, carotenoids in beet juice can improve the quality, shine and thickness of the hair. They assist in circulation of blood in hair follicles and with that promote hair growth. A natural remedy to prevent hair loss is mixing ginger with beet juice and applying it on the scalp.

Recipes

Chapter # 1: Beetroot and Walnut Salad

Makes: 6 serving

Prep time: 20 minutes

Cooking time: 45 minutes

Ingredients:

- 2 bunches baby beetroot
- 140 g caster sugar
- 55 g walnut halves
- Olive oil, for greasing
- 2 bunches rocket leaves
- ½ teaspoon sea salt
- 80 g goat's cheese
- 60 ml extra virgin oil
- 1 tablespoon red wine vinegar

Directions:

First, preheat the oven to 200 degrees Celsius. Then use a fork to prick the beetroots and place them on a baking tray and bake for 45 minutes. After they are done set them aside to cool, then peel and halve. While the beetroots are baking, line a baking tray with baking paper and place a wire rack brushed with olive oil on it. Place the sugar in a nonstick pan over medium heat and cook without stirring but tilting the pan, for four minutes until the sugar melts. Stir in the walnuts and pour them onto the rack. Separate the walnuts and sprinkle some salt. Put this aside for 30 minutes. Combine the rocket leaves and beetroots in a bowl and top it with goat cheese plus the walnuts. Combine the oil and vinegar in a jug and drizzle over the product.

Chapter # 2: Tandoori Cutlets with Beetroot Raita

Makes: 4 serving

Prep time: 15 minutes

Cooking time: 10 minutes

Ingredients:

- ¼ cup tandoori paste
- ¼ cup yogurt
- 12 lamb cutlets
- 2 teaspoons grated ginger
- 2 Lebanese cucumbers (cut into ribbons)
- 2 carrots (cut into ribbons)
- 1 cup coriander leaves
- 1 tablespoon lemon juice
- Steamed *SunRice* Basmati Rice

For Beetroot Raita:

- 2 teaspoons cumin seeds
- 1 cup natural yogurt
- 1 teaspoon black mustard seeds
- 1 medium beetroot, peeled and grated
- 1/3 cup desiccated coconut

Directions:

Combine the tandoori paste, ginger and yogurt in a large bowl, either glass or ceramic. Add the lamb and coat it with the mixture. Cover with a plastic wrap and place it in the fridge for an hour so it can marinate.

To make the Raita, place the mustard and cumin seeds in a frying pan over medium heat. Cook while tossing for a minute and then combine the mustard and cumin seeds, beetroot, yogurt and coconut in a small bowl.

Heat a large frying pan over medium-intensity heat and add the cutlets, cooking them for 2-3 minutes each side or until cooked to your liking. Transfer to a plate and cover it with foil. Put aside for five minutes. Finally combine the carrot, lemon juice, cucumber and coriander leaves in a bowl and divide them among many plates. Top the lamb cutlets and serve with Raita and steamed rice.

Chapter # 3: Beetroot Hummus

Makes: 2 cups

Prep time: 10 minutes

Ingredients:

- 450 g chopped and drained, canned beetroot
- 400 g rinsed and drained, canned chickpeas
- 2 garlic cloves, chopped
- 1 tablespoon lemon juice
- 1 tablespoon sesame paste
- 2 tablespoons olive oil
- Warmed Turkish bread

Directions:

Place the chickpeas, garlic, beetroot, sesame paste and lemon juice in a food processor and whiz to make a paste. While the motor is running, add oil until a thick & smooth mixture is obtained. Season well and serve with Turkish bread.

Conclusion

Beetroot has undoubtedly proven itself one of the top contenders in the race for vegetable supremacy. It has health-promoting compounds ranging from the vital antioxidants to the unique phytonutrients, all there to help bring the body to its best shape. Pharmaceutical companies have already started extraction of many worthy nutrients from the taproot and have incorporated them in their drugs that range from anti-inflammatories to stamina-boosters for athletes. All in all, whether you roast it, blend it, or drink its juice, beetroot would always be there for you with its low fat, vitamin & mineral rich content and purple hue to help you get back on your feet!

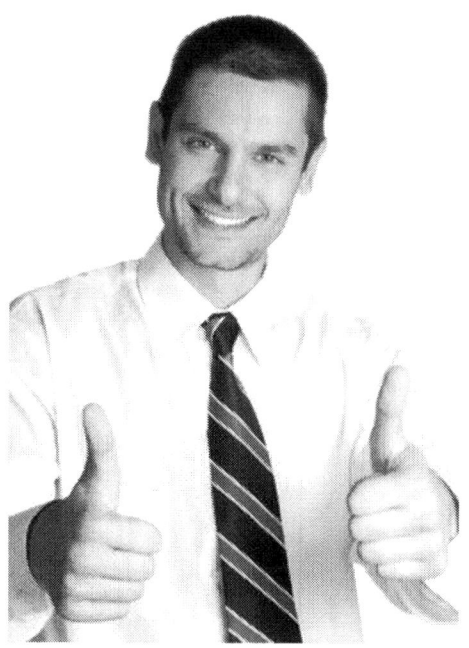

References

http://www.123rf.com/photo_10014309_fresh-red-beet-on-a-white-background.html?term=beetroot

http://www.123rf.com/photo_27778199_fresh-juice-of-red-beets-on-white.html?term=beetroot%20health

http://www.123rf.com/photo_4659885_fresh-spinach-and-beetroot-juice-isolated-white-background.html?term=beetroot

http://www.123rf.com/photo_20235889_brain-aging-and-memory-loss-due-to-dementia-and-alzheimer.html?term=dementia

http://www.fotolia.com/id/37121015

http://www.fotolia.com/id/41000500

http://www.fotolia.com/id/51802921

http://www.fotolia.com/id/54507728

http://www.fotolia.com/id/51102457

Author Bio

Muhammad Usman is a distinguished medical graduate of Allama iqbal medical college (AIMC). He is a professional writer who has been in the field for more than 4 years. During this time he has produced 10,000+ articles, blogs and eBooks on various niches related to diseases, health, fitness, nutrition and well-being. He is a regular contributor to several journals related to medicine and surgery. He is the editor of several journals and newspapers.

Check out some of the other JD-Biz Publishing books

Gardening Series on Amazon

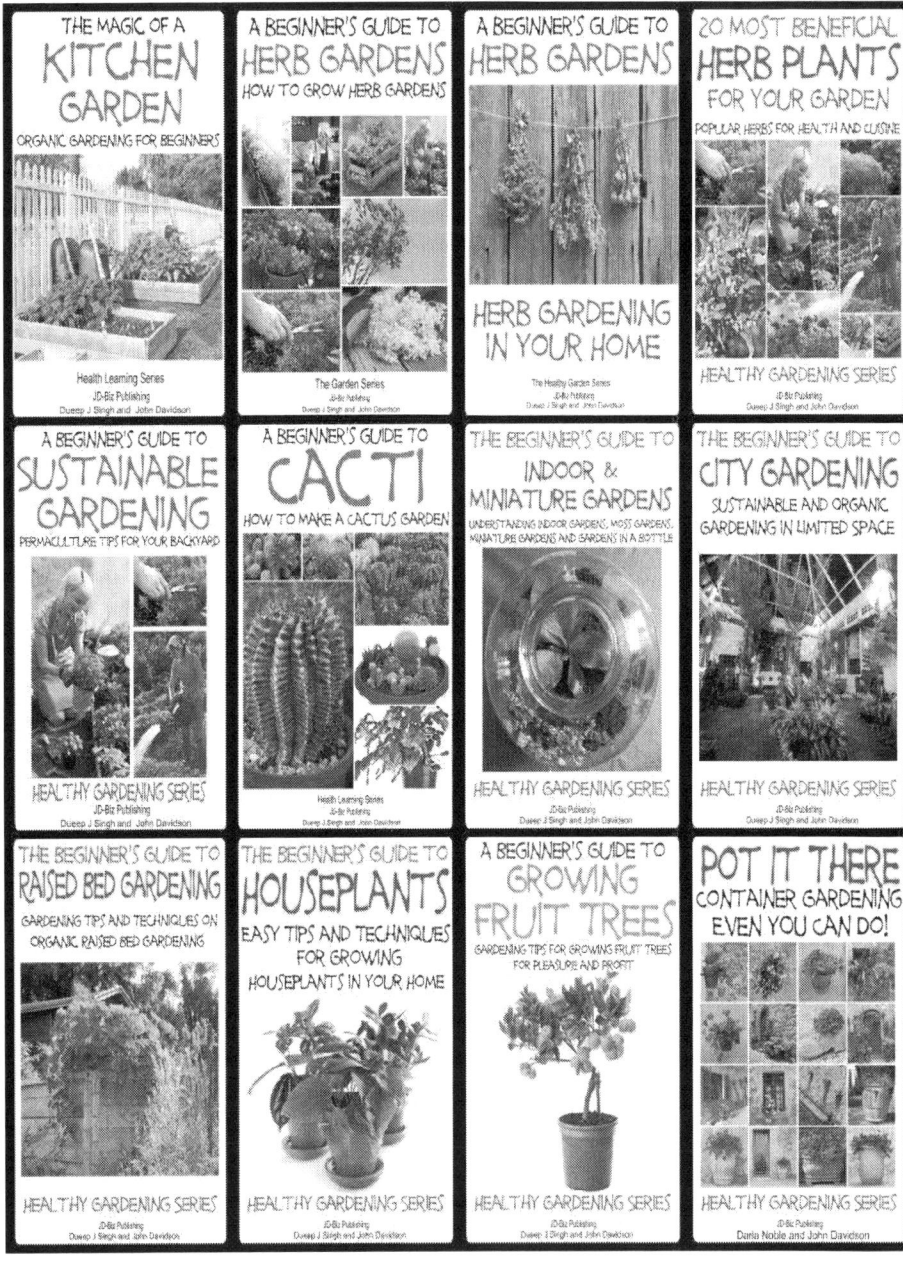

Health Learning Series

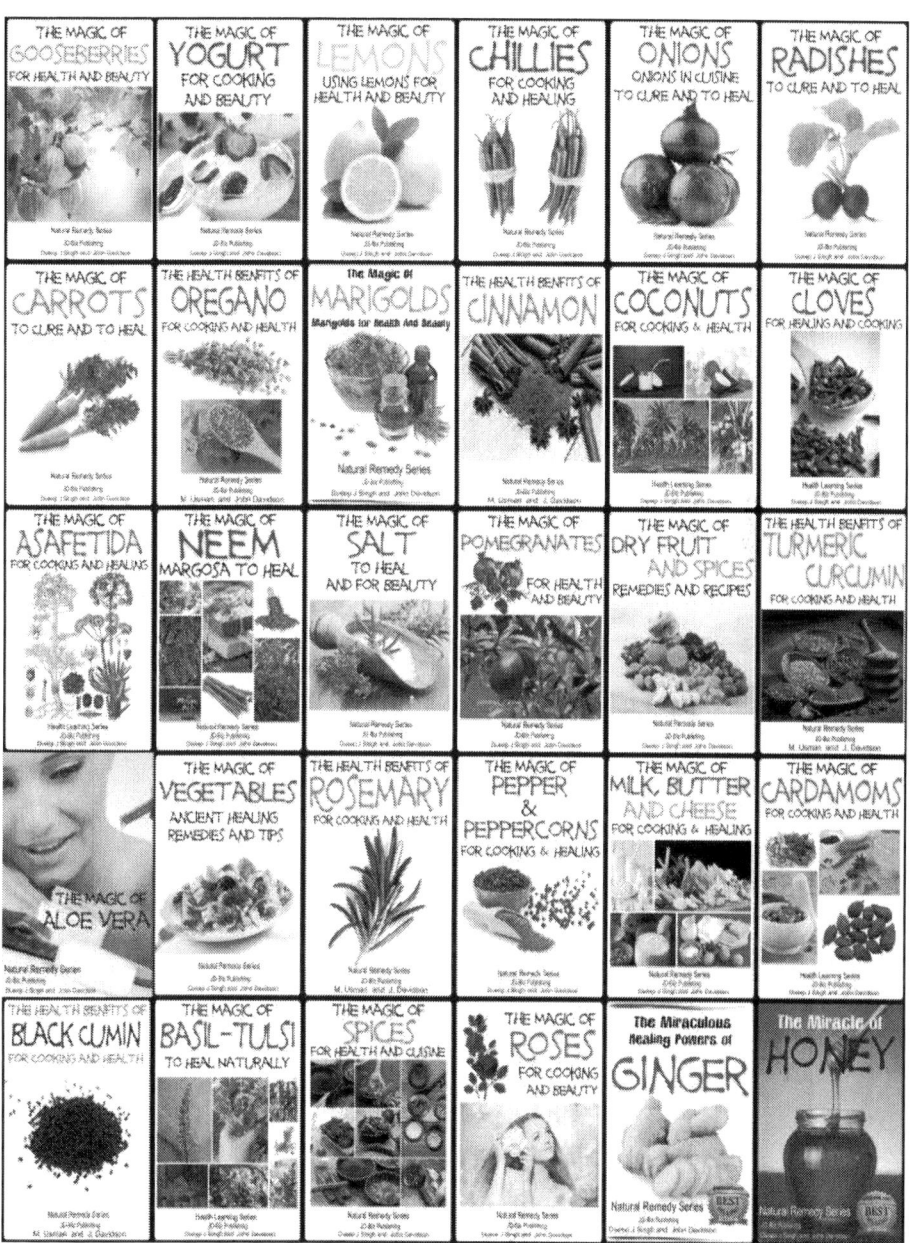

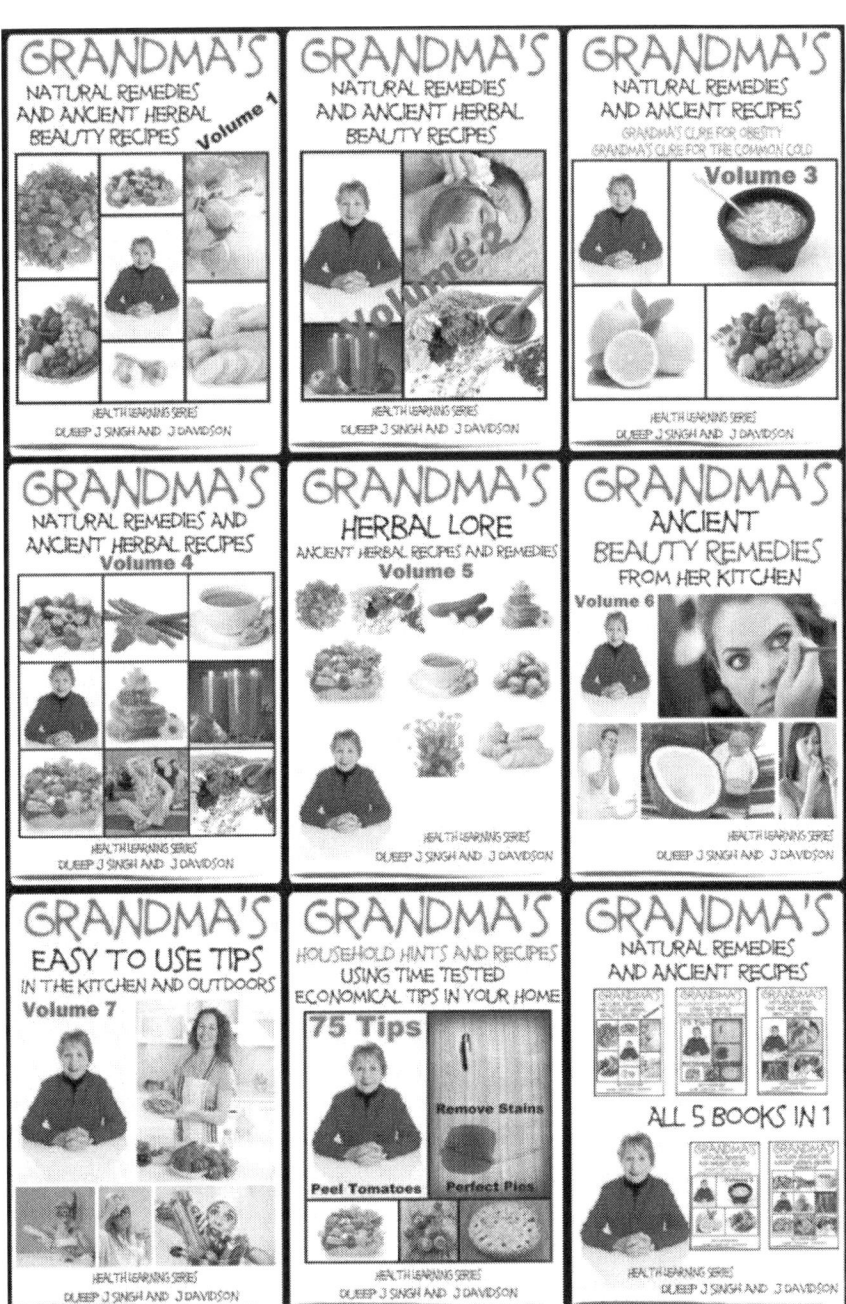

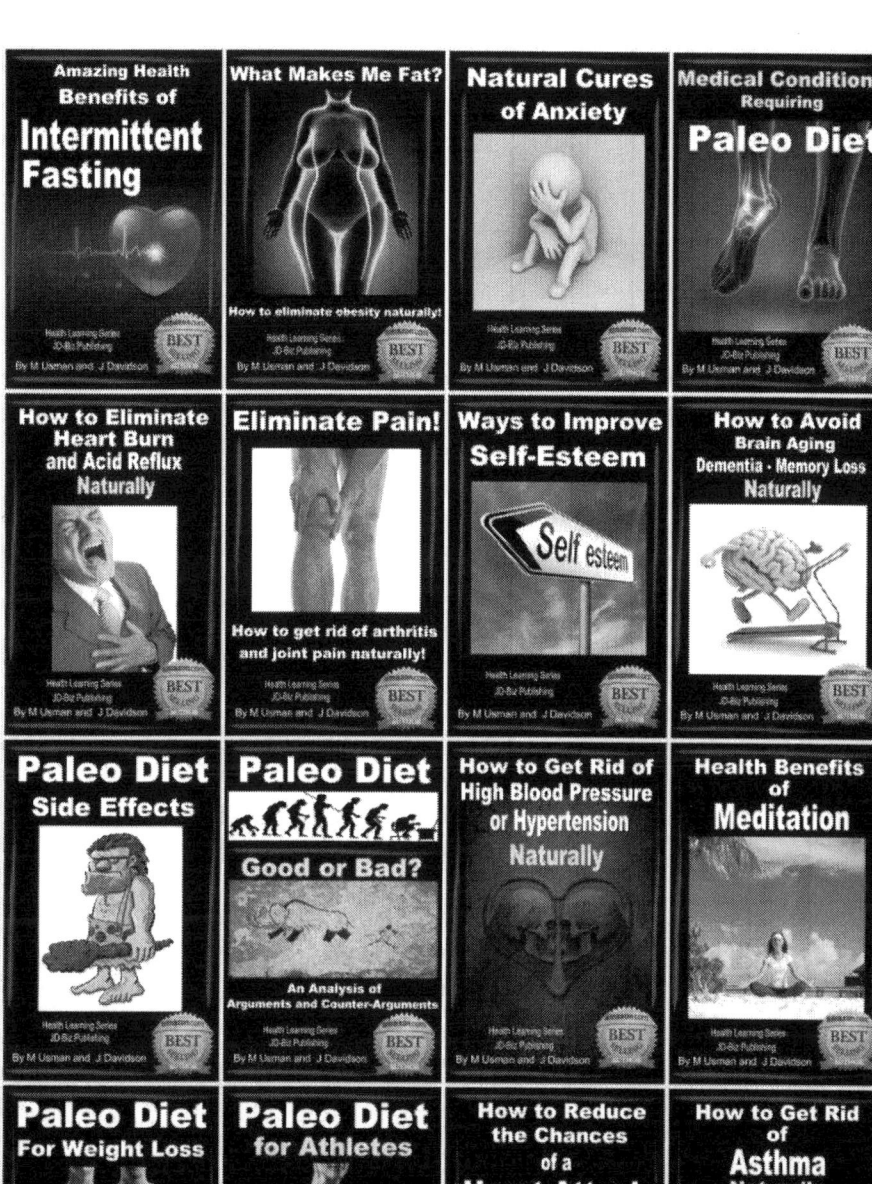

Amazing Animal Book Series

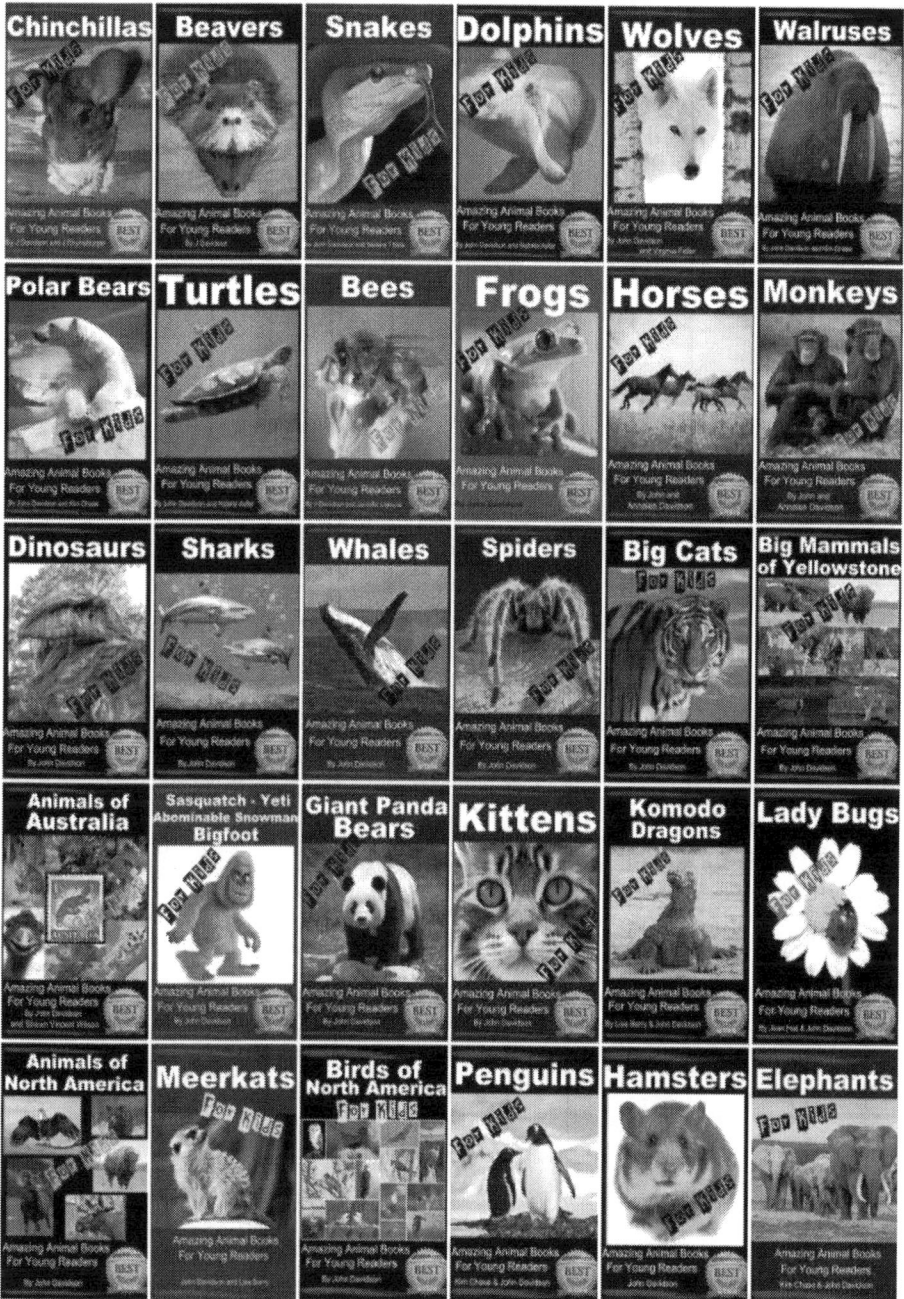

Learn To Draw Series

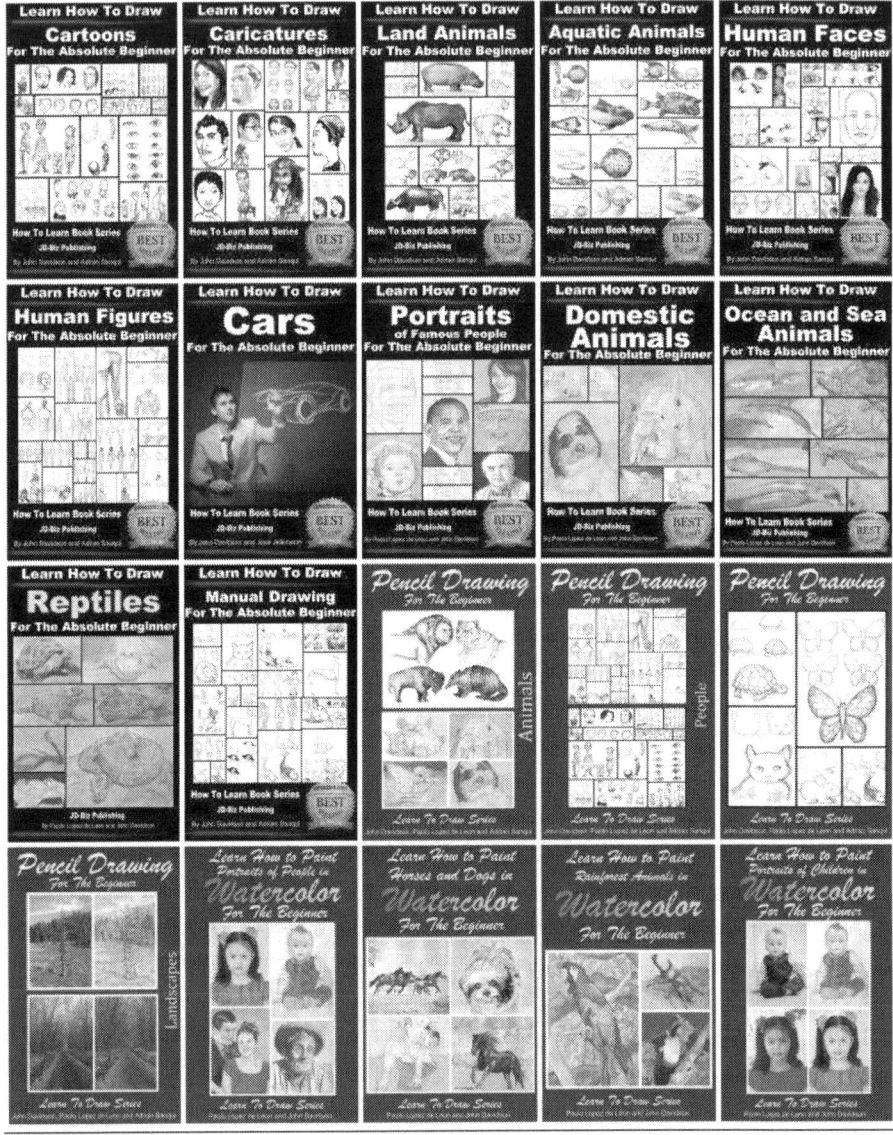

How to Build and Plan Books

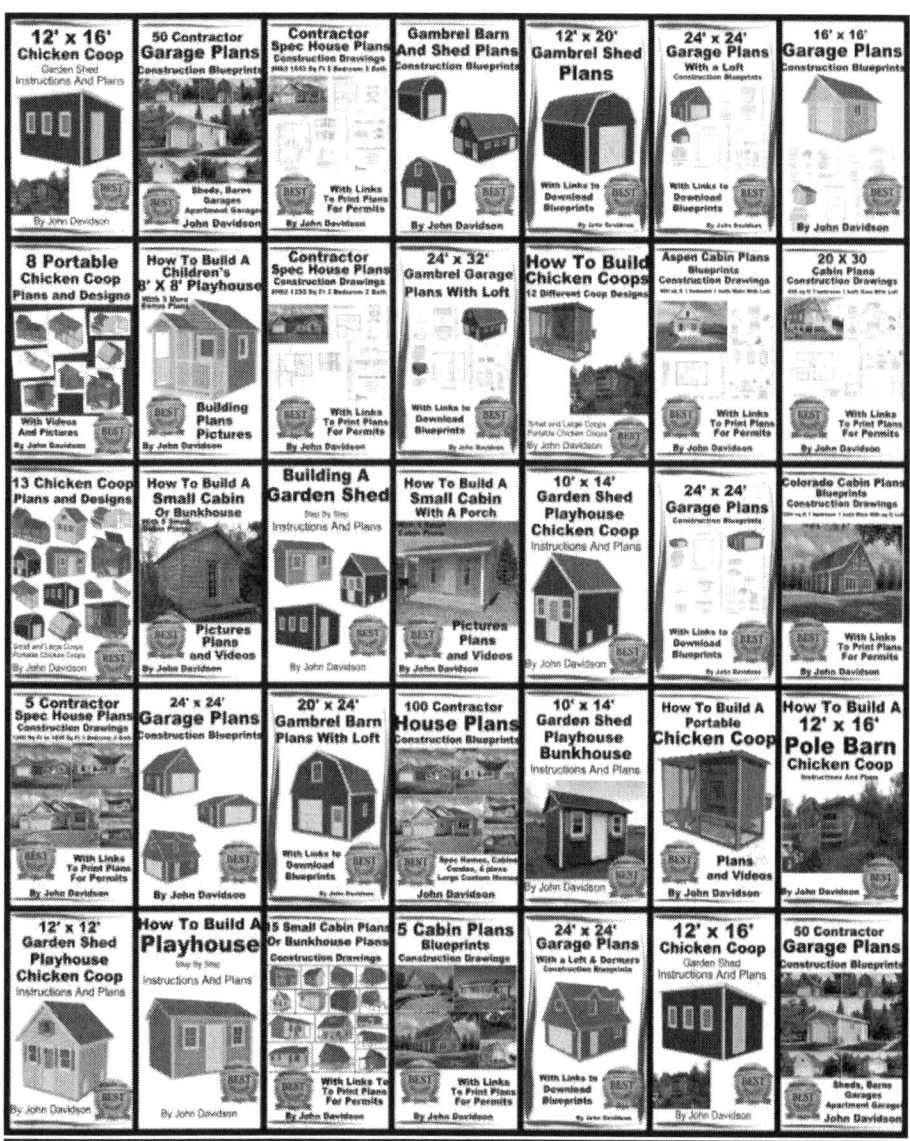

Entrepreneur Book Series

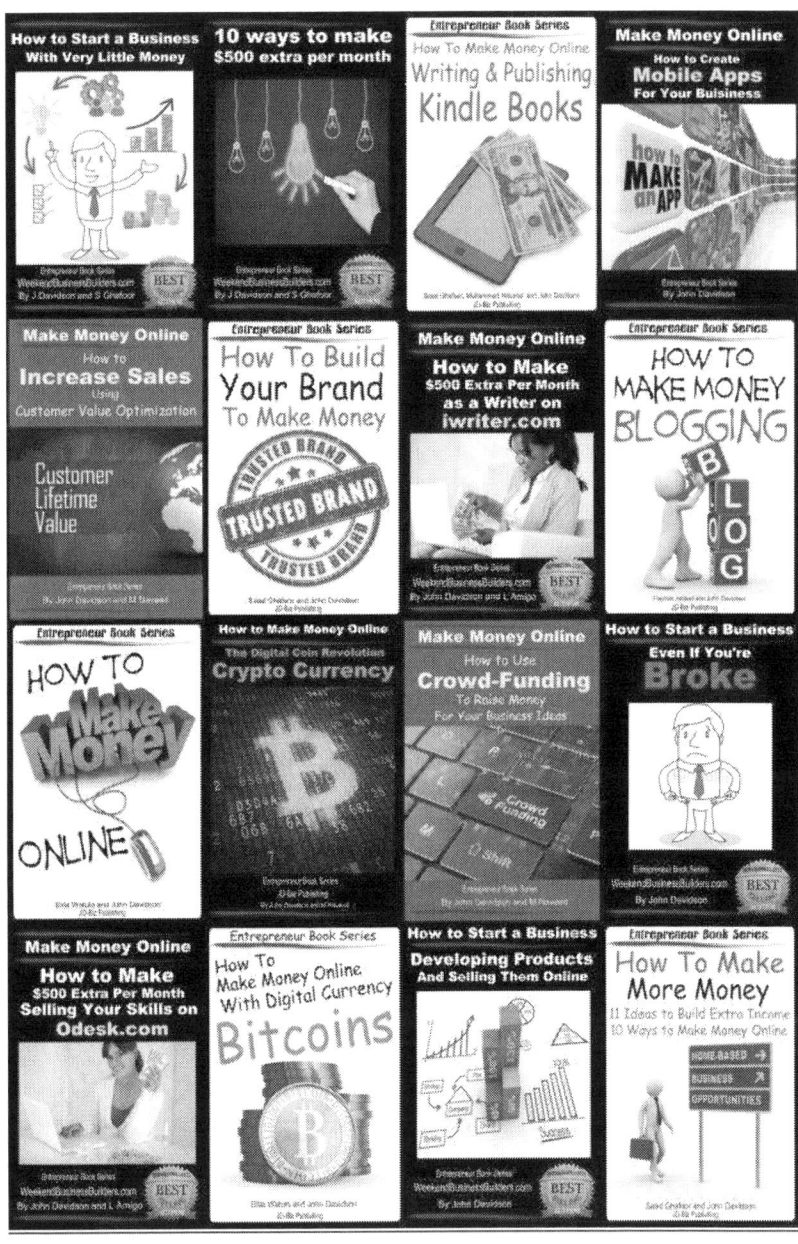

Our books are available at

1. Amazon.com
2. Barnes and Noble
3. Itunes
4. Kobo
5. Smashwords
6. Google Play Books

This book is published by

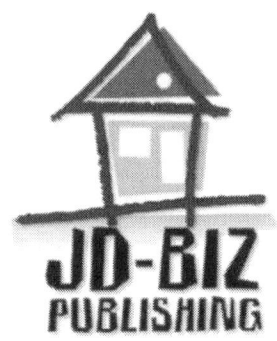

JD-Biz Corp

P O Box 374

Mendon, Utah 84325

http://www.jd-biz.com/

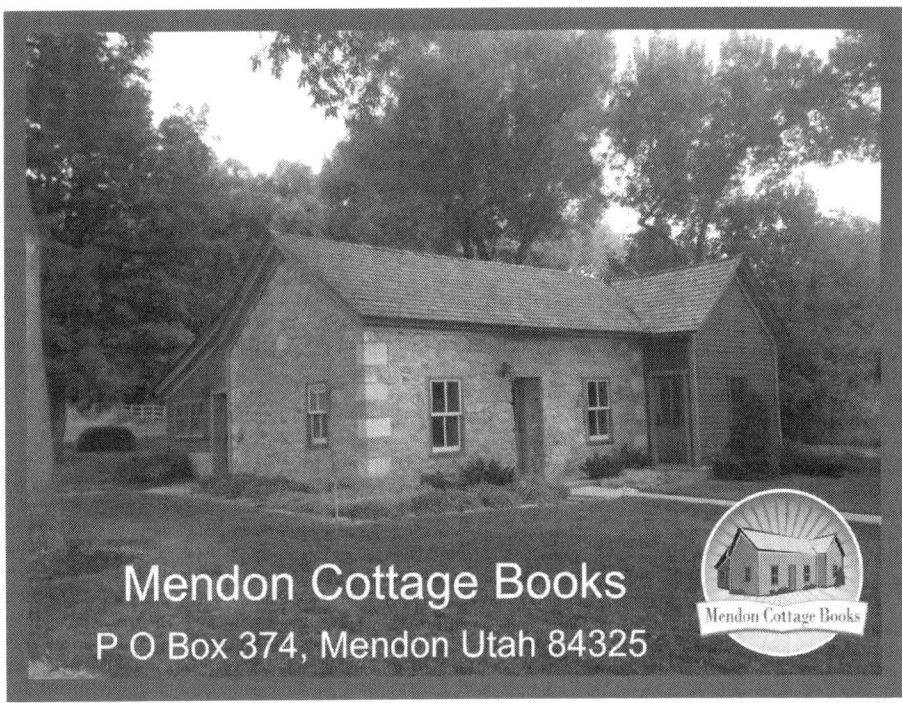

Printed in Great Britain
by Amazon